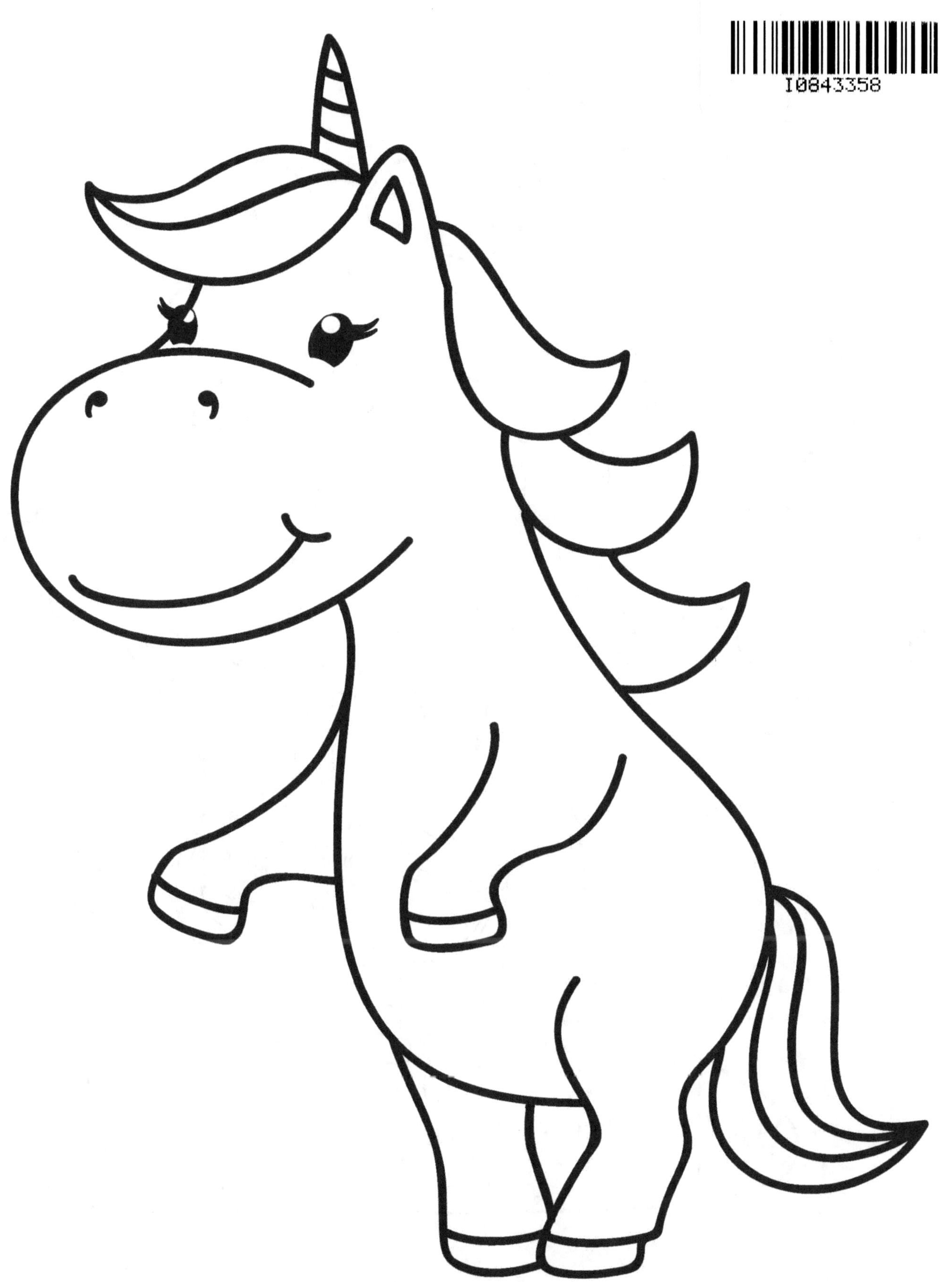

HI! MY NAME IS DAISY

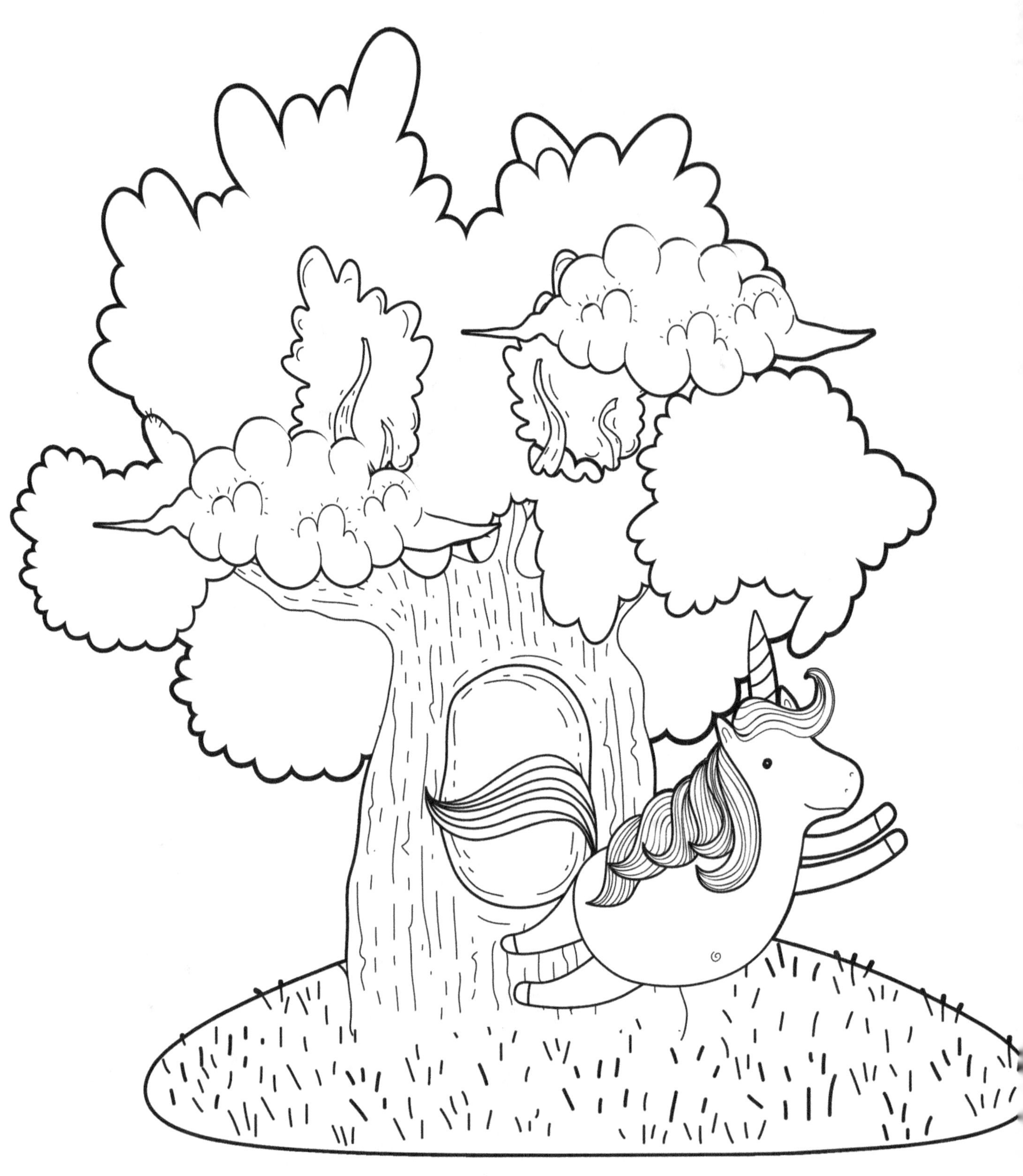

I LIVE IN THE MAGIC FOREST

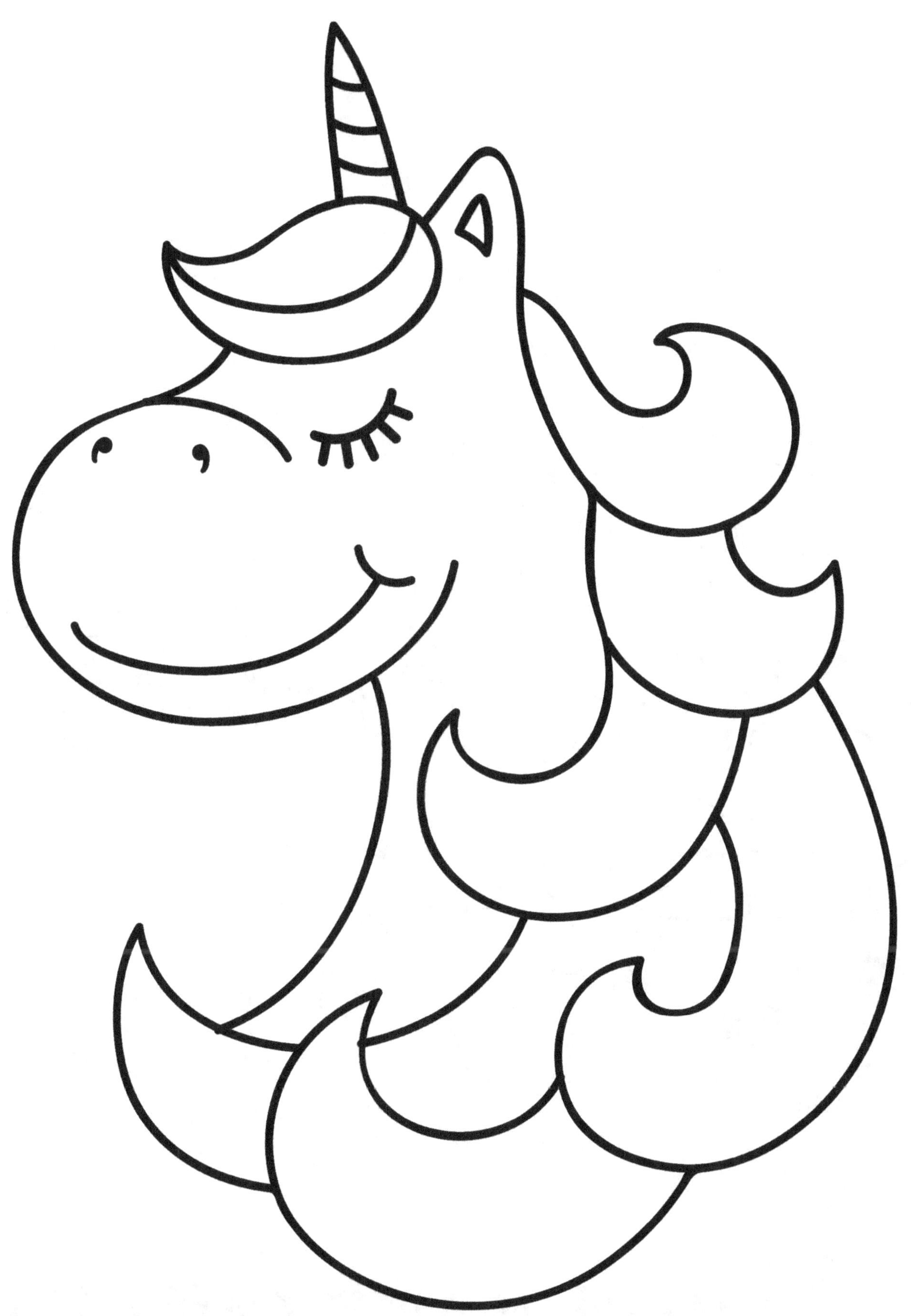

I HAVE TYPE 1 DIABETES

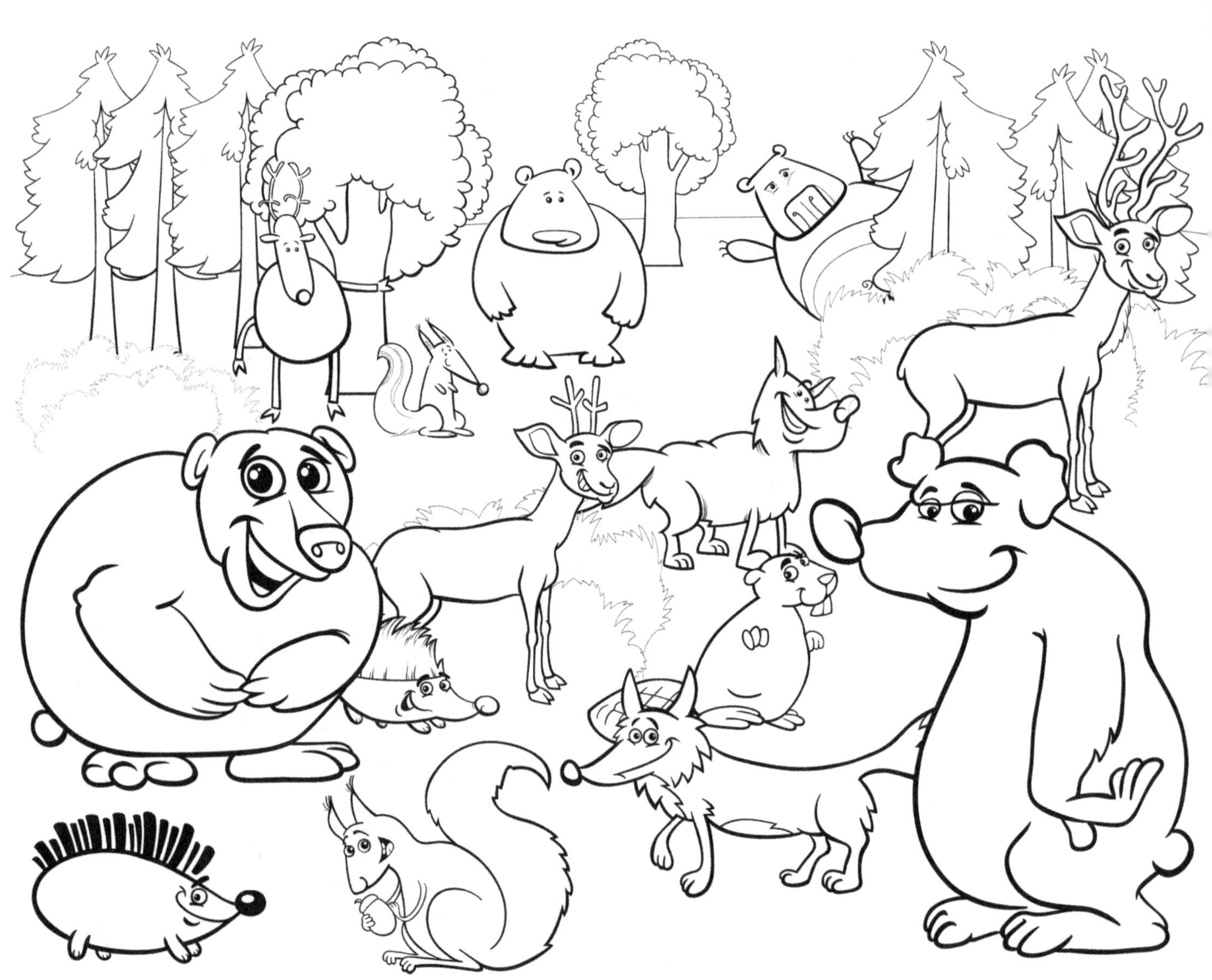

I HAVE MANY FRIENDS BUT NONE WITH DIABETES.

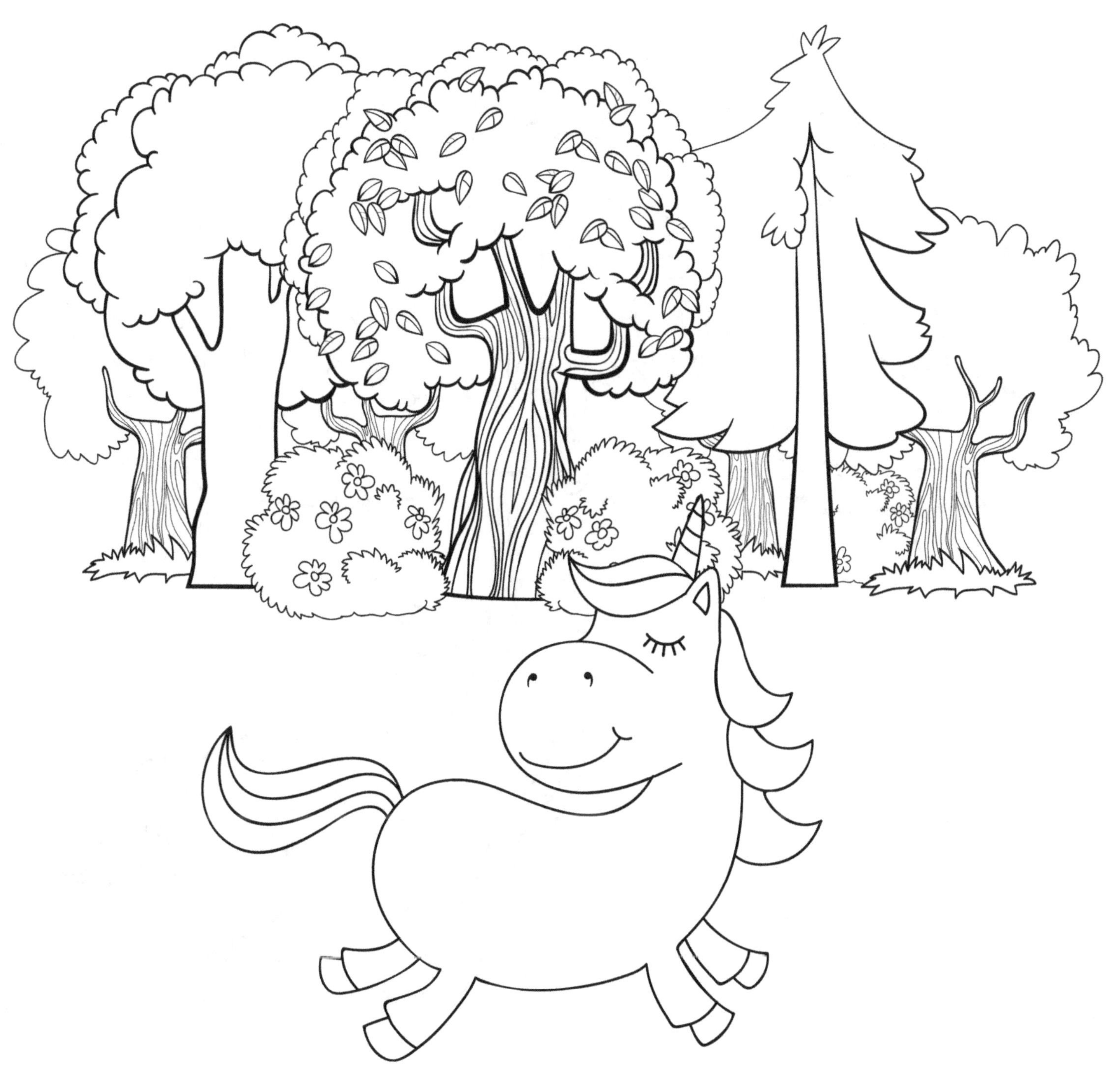

SO I THOUGHT I WOULD FIND A FRIEND LIKE ME!

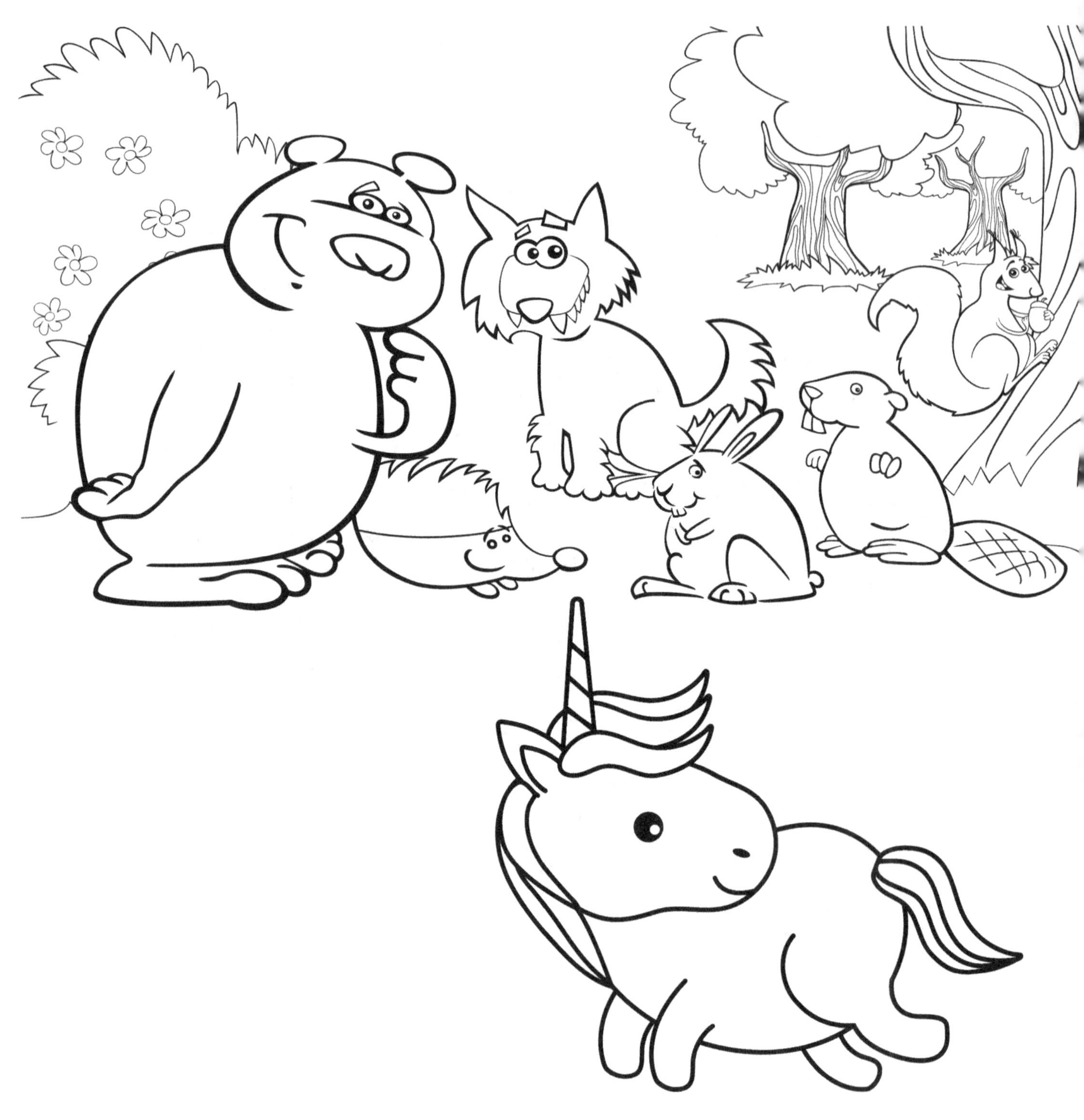

I LOOKED ALL OVER THE FOREST....

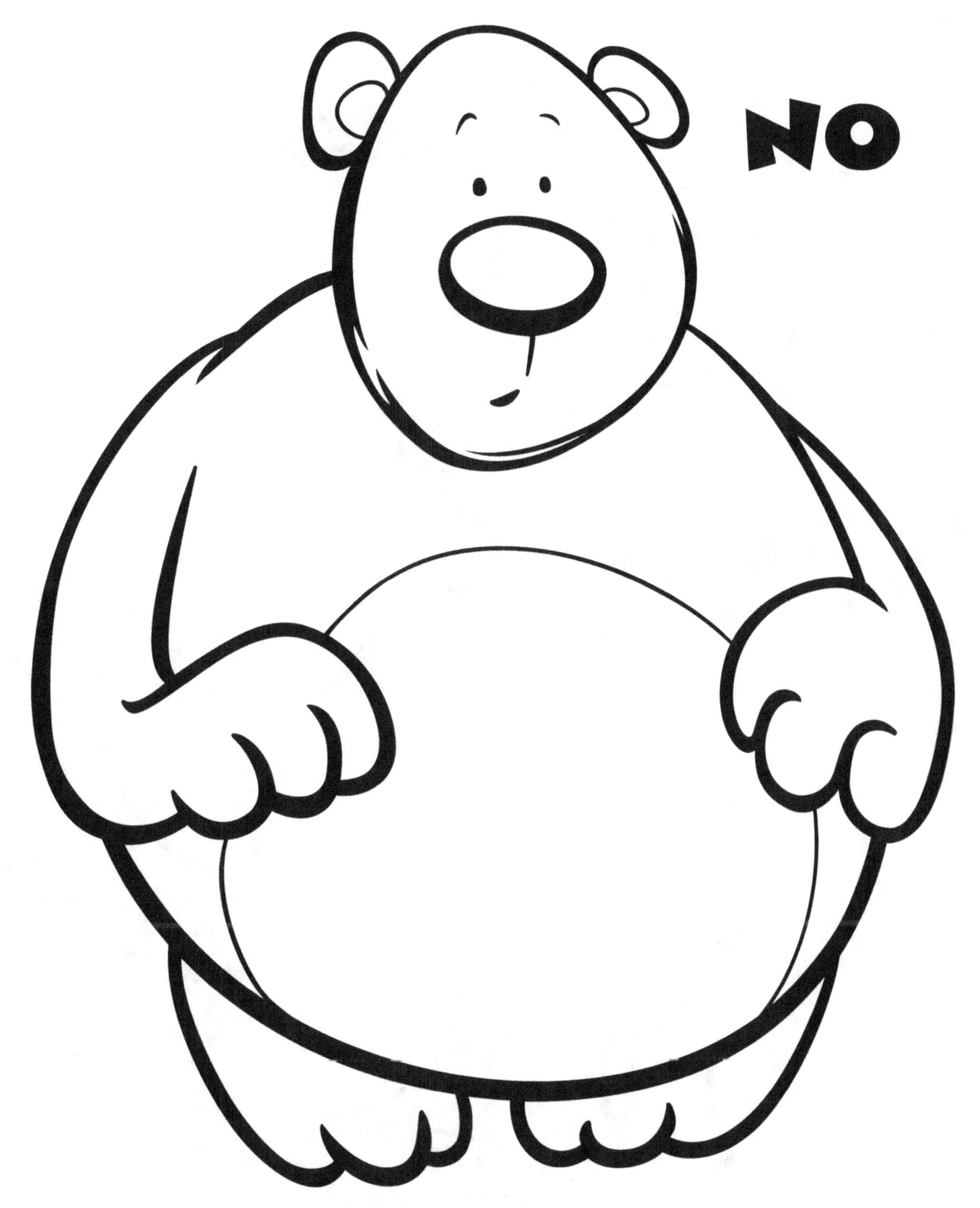

ARE YOU A TYPE 1 DIABETIC?

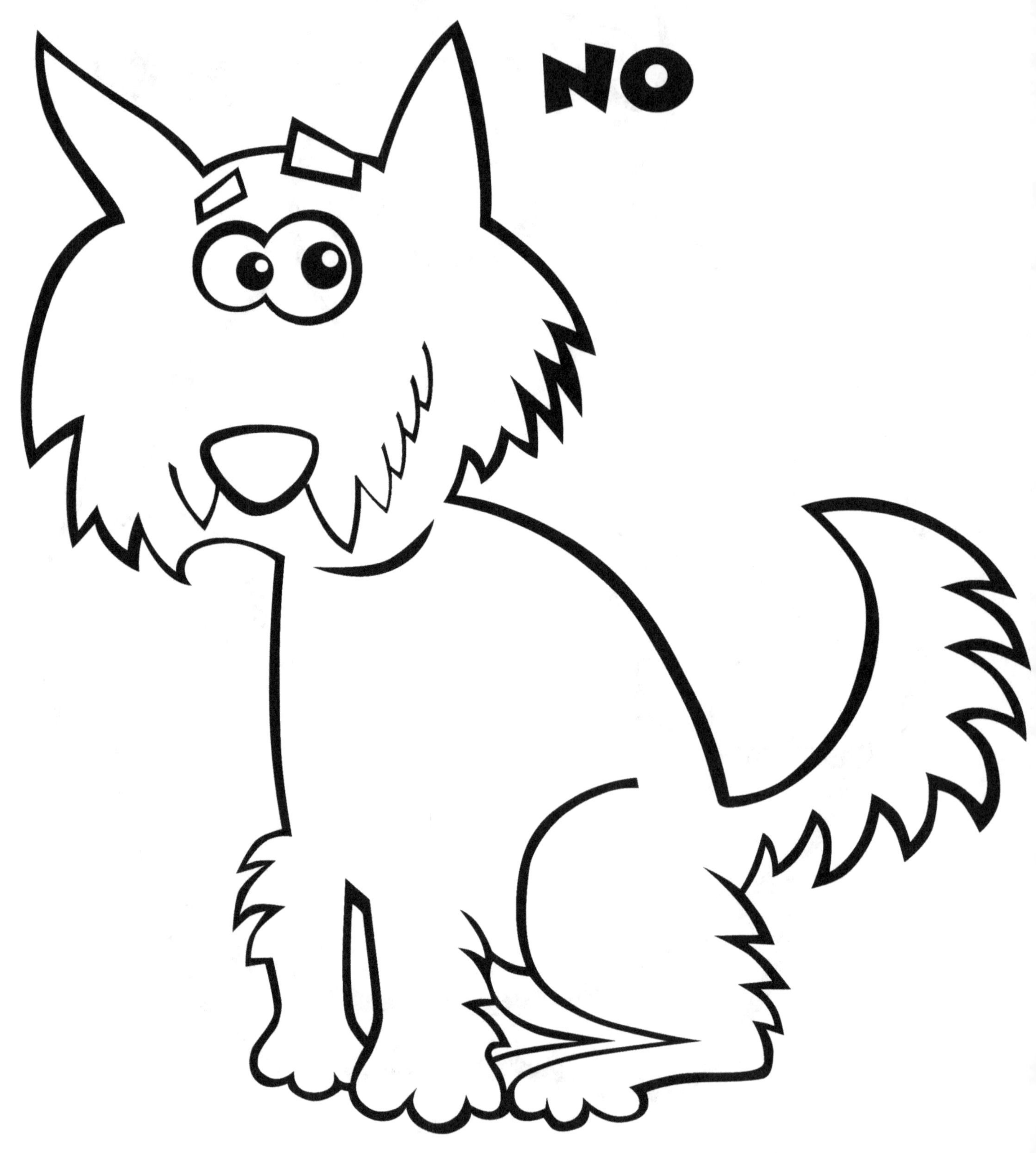

ARE YOU A TYPE 1 DIABETIC?

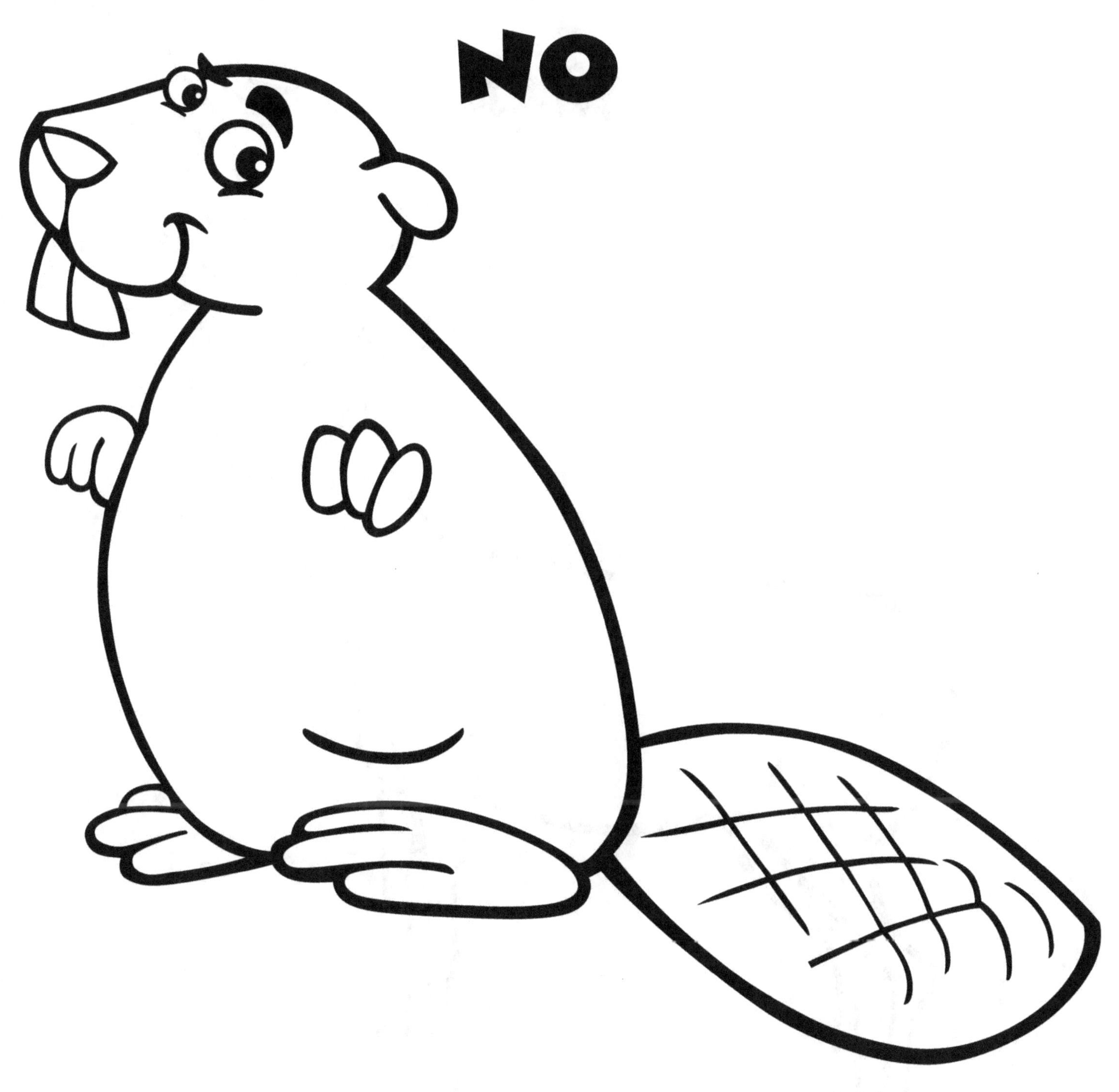

ARE YOU A TYPE 1 DIABETIC?

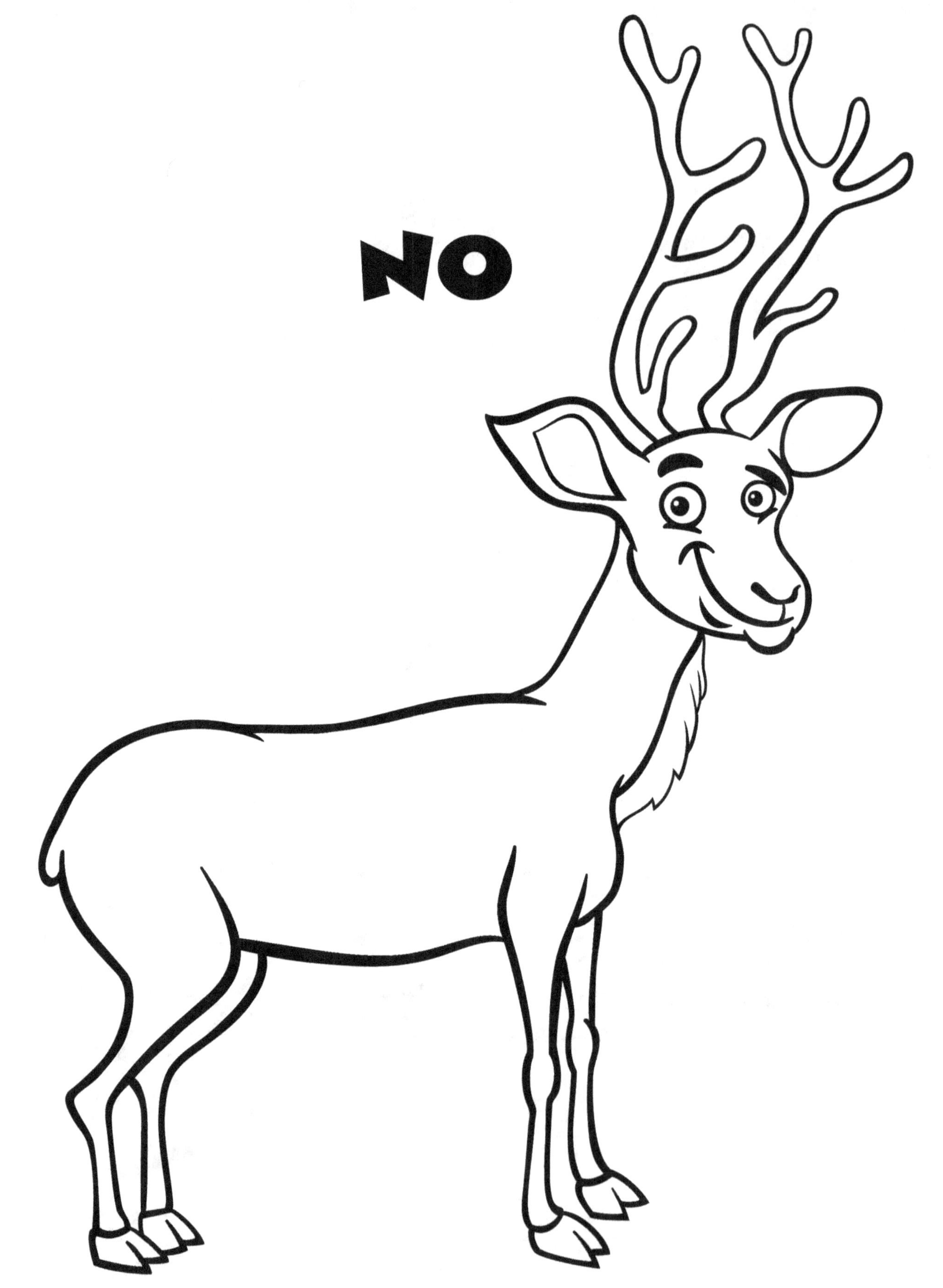

NO
ARE YOU A TYPE 1 DIABETIC?

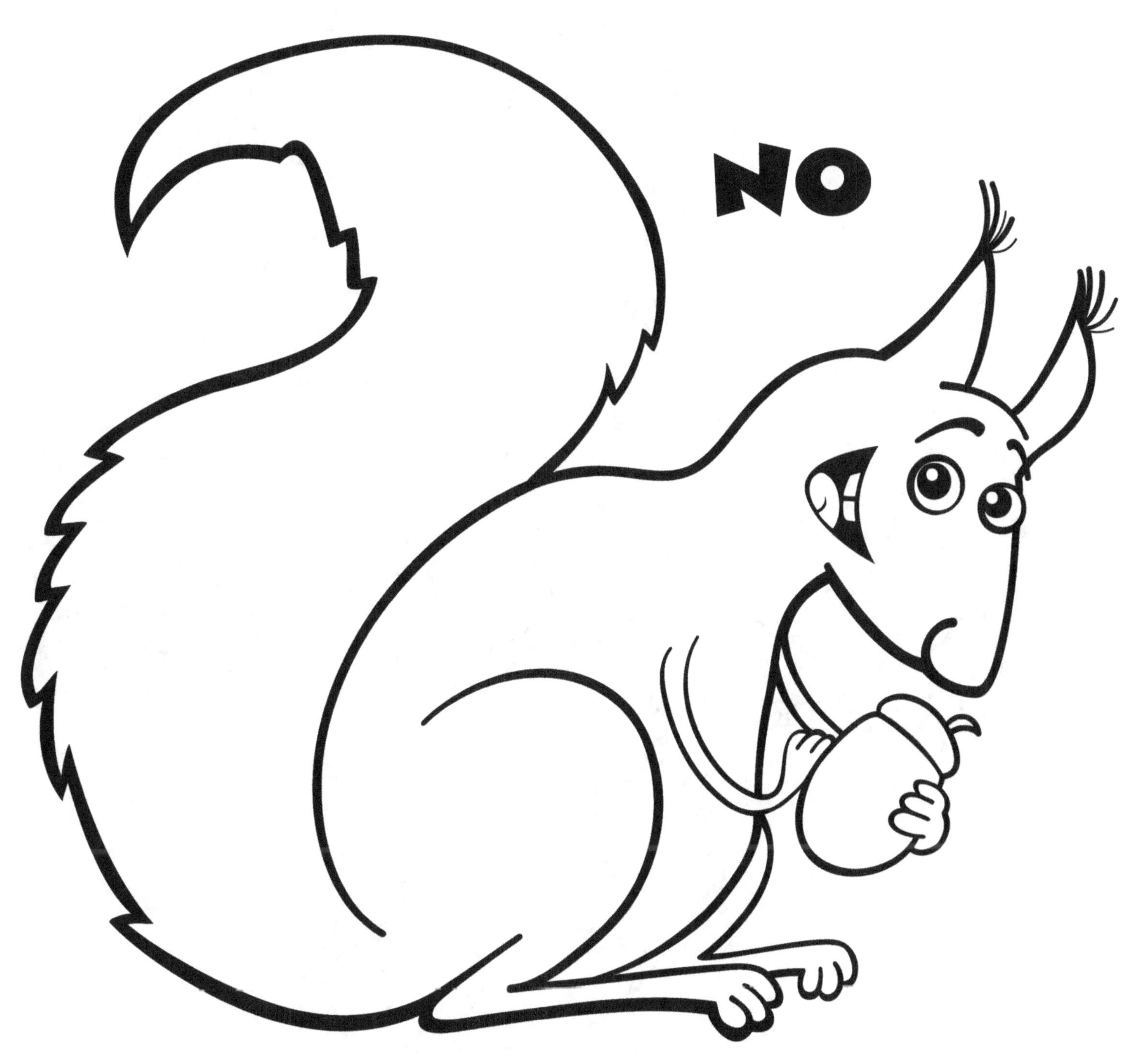

ARE YOU A TYPE 1 DIABETIC?

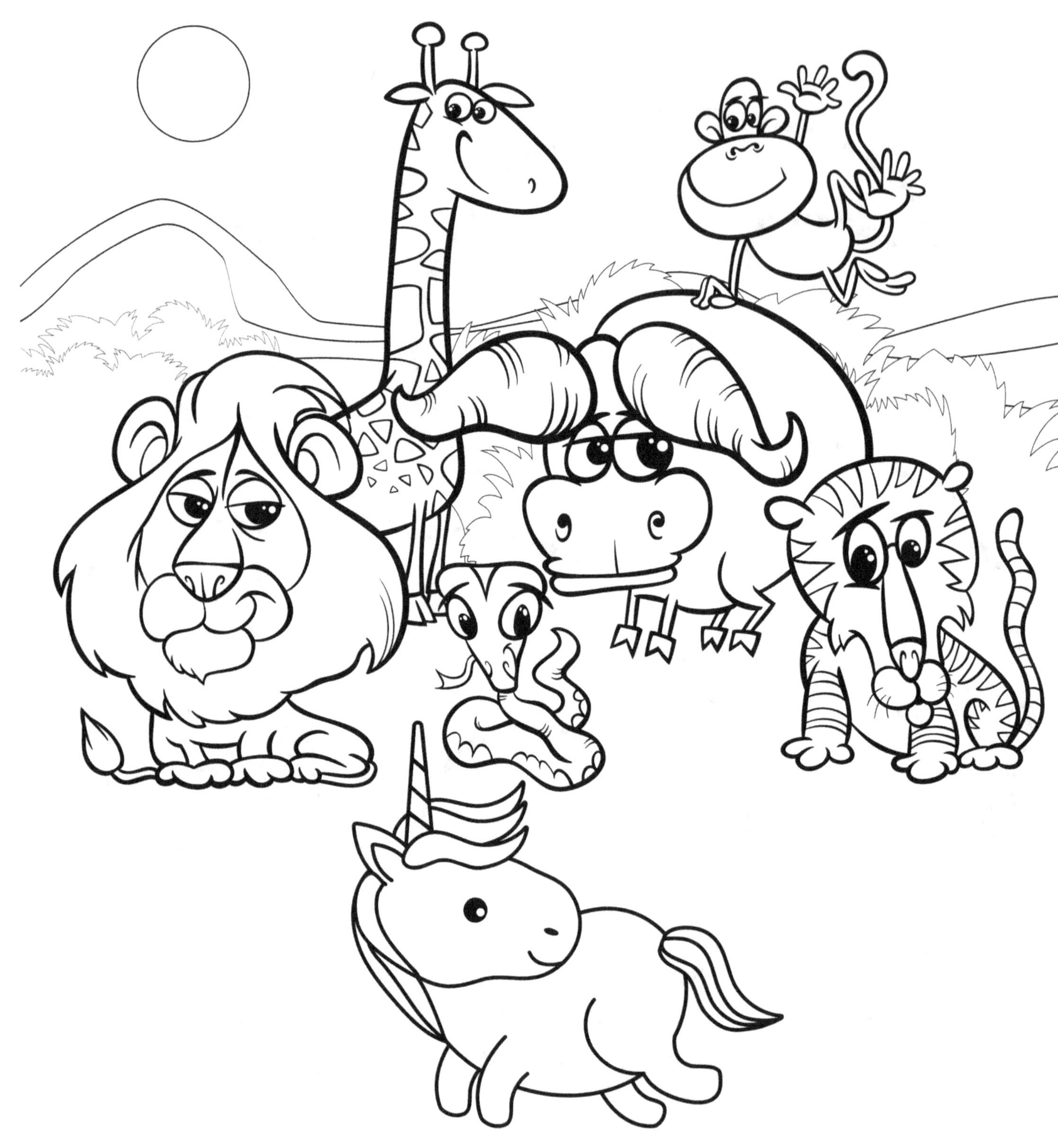

I LOOKED ALL OVER THE JUNGLE....

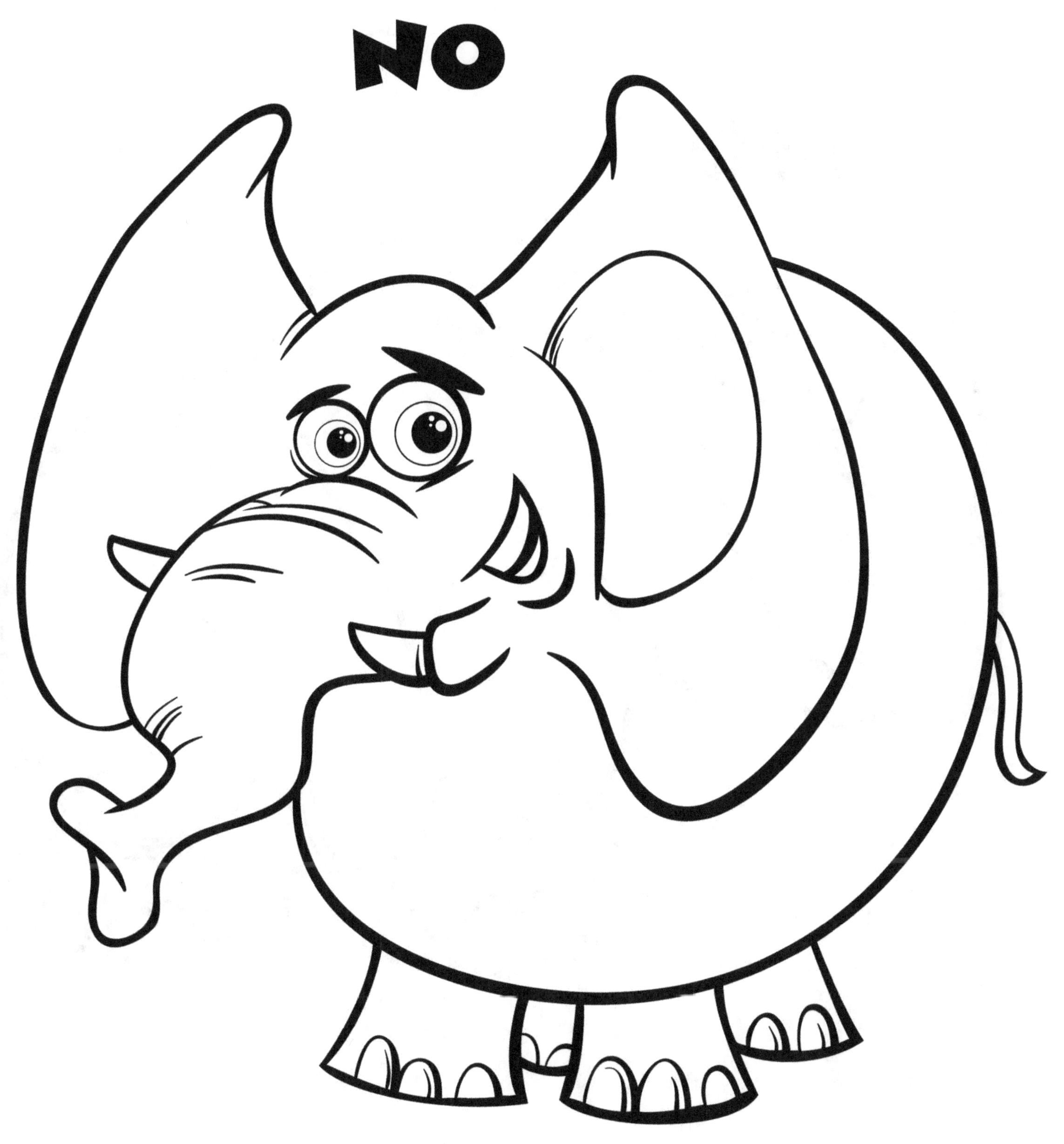

ARE YOU A TYPE 1 DIABETIC?

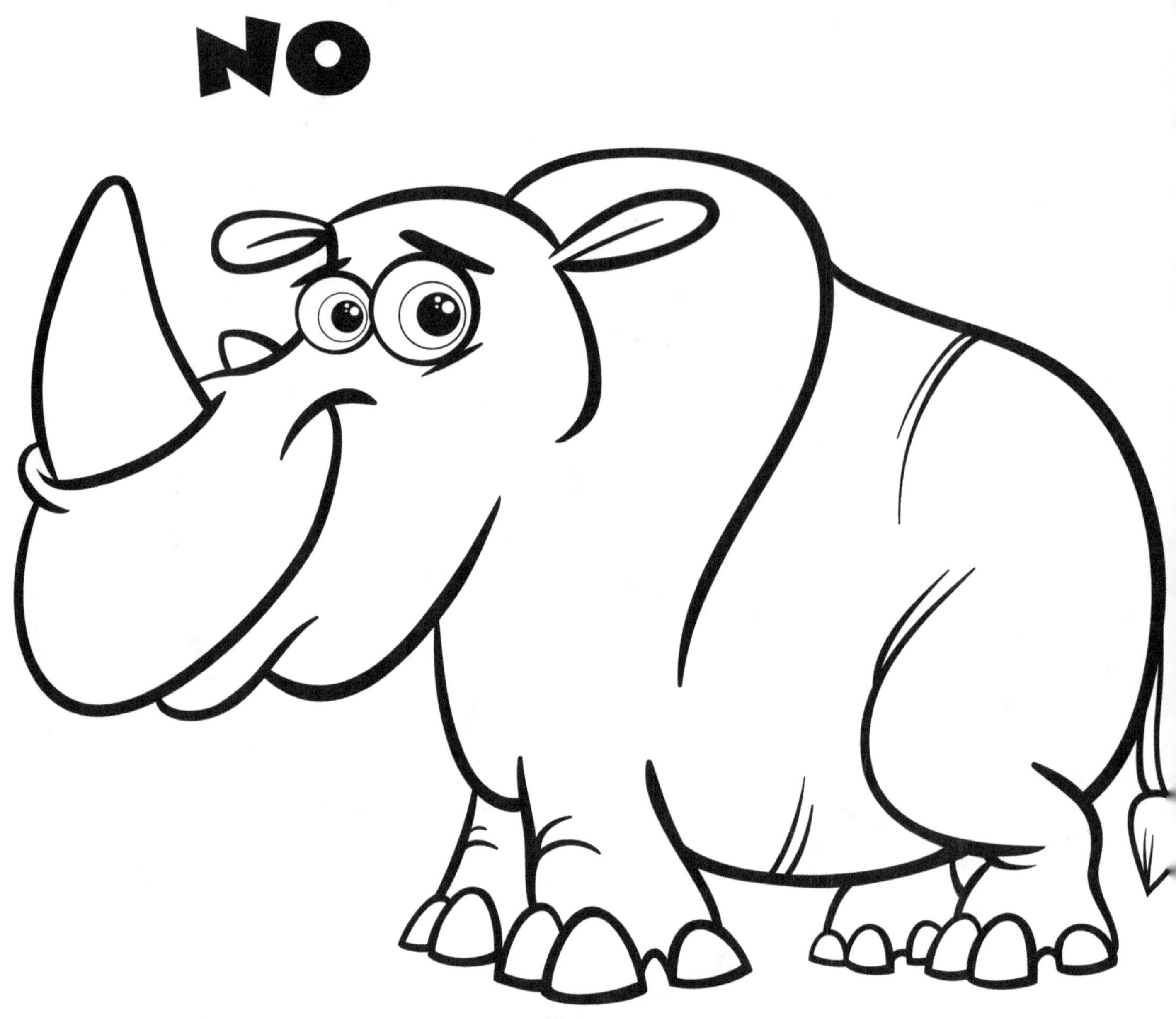

ARE YOU A TYPE 1 DIABETIC.

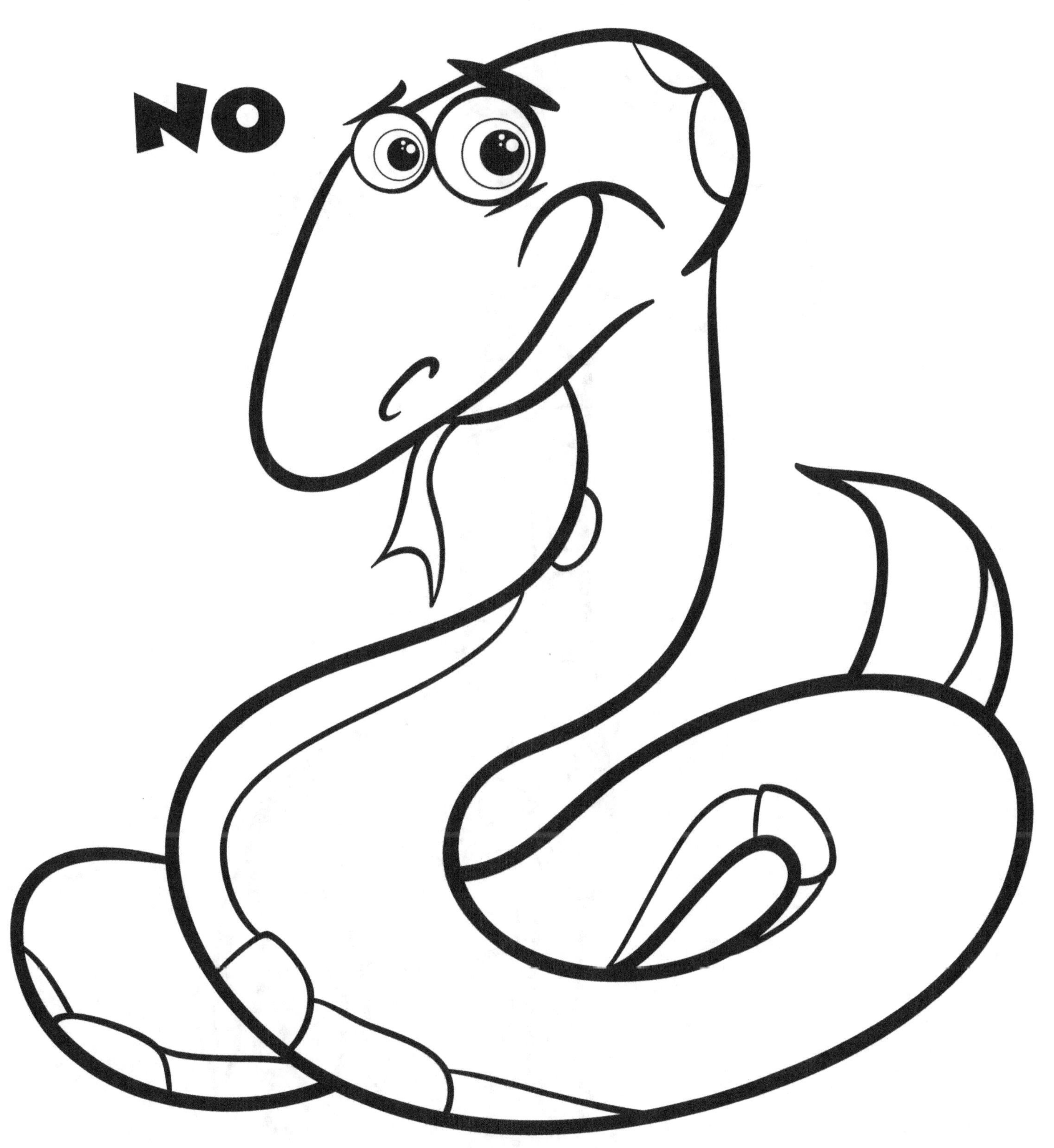

NO
ARE YOU A TYPE 1 DIABETIC?

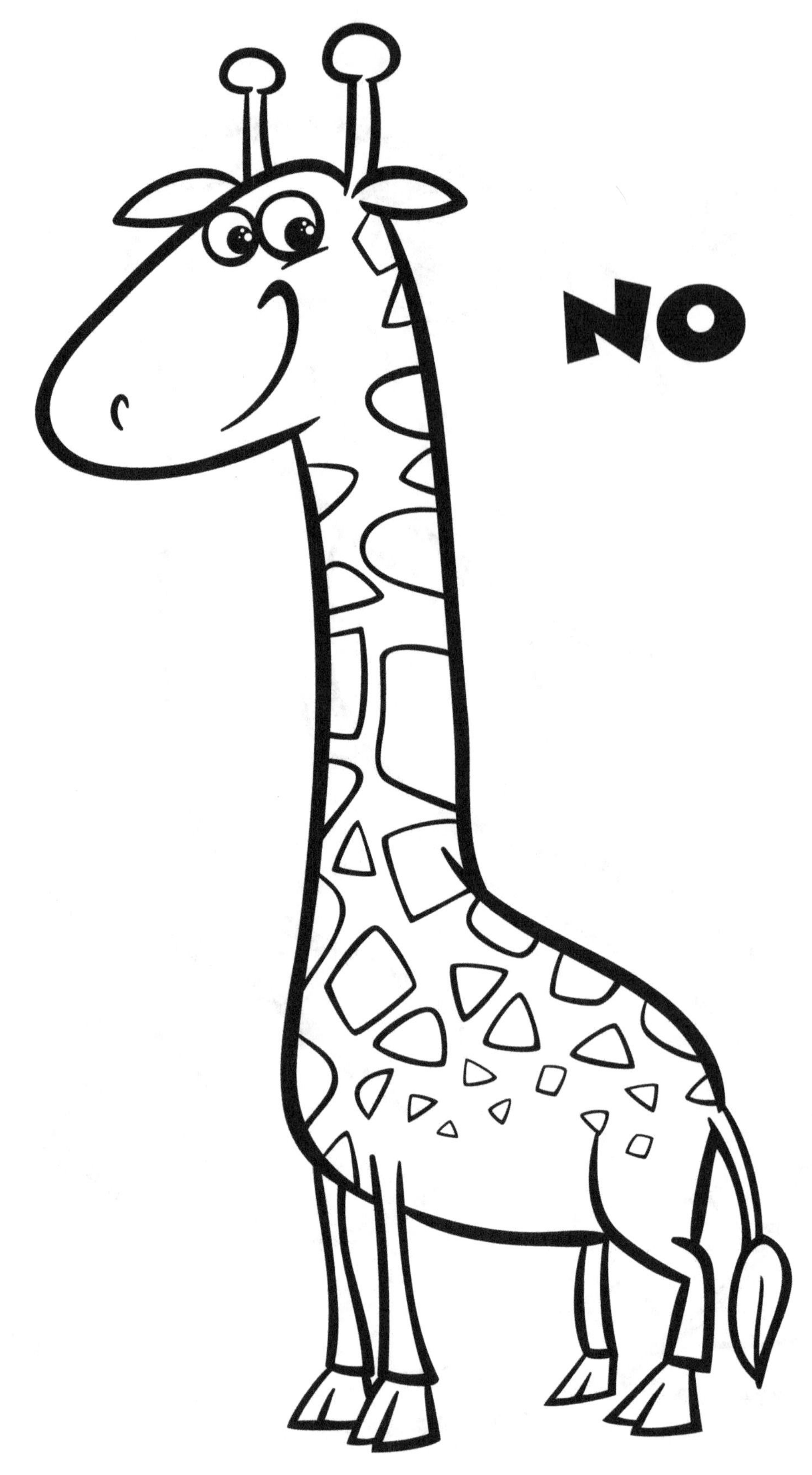

NO
ARE YOU A TYPE 1 DIABETIC?

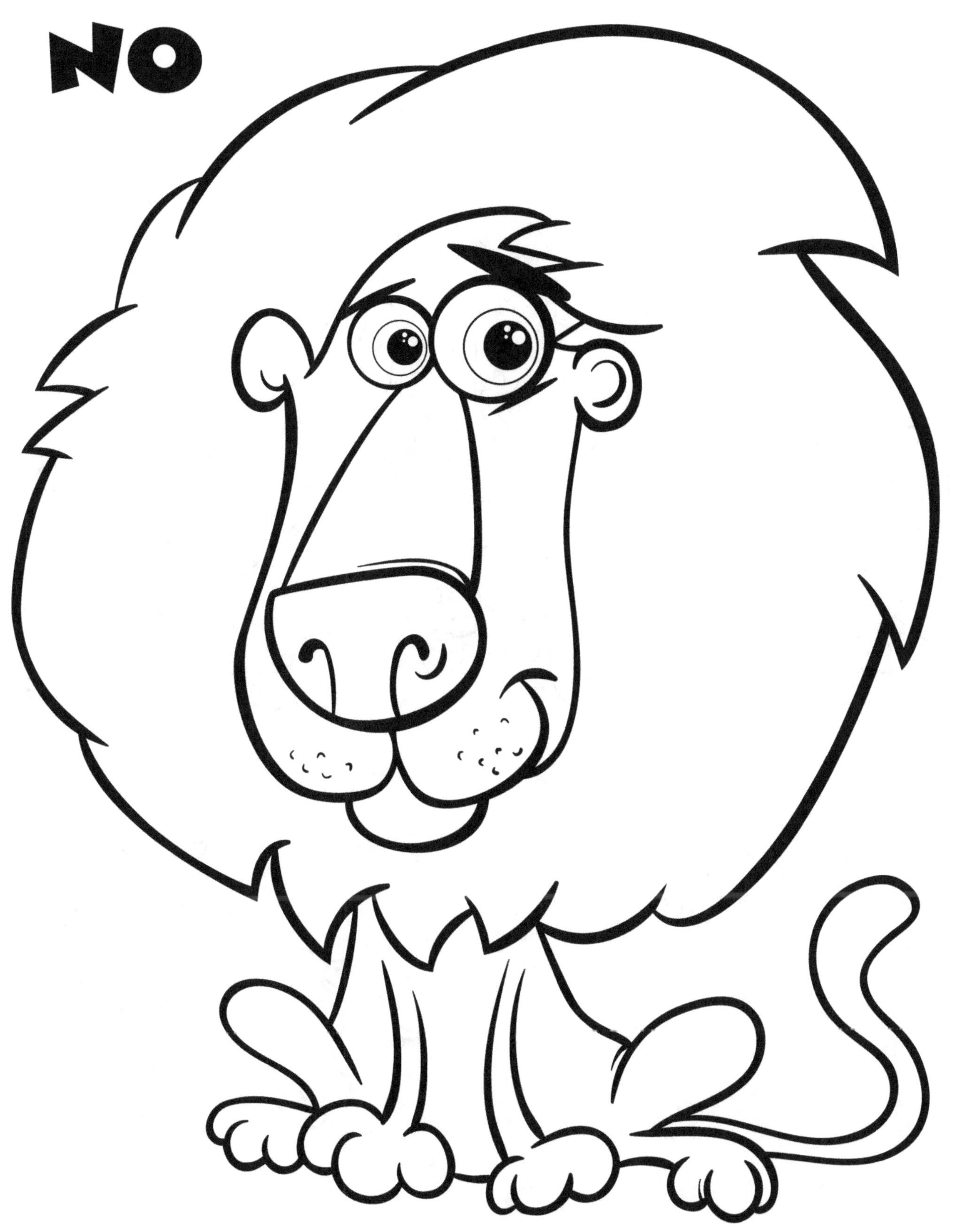

NO
ARE YOU A TYPE 1 DIABETIC?

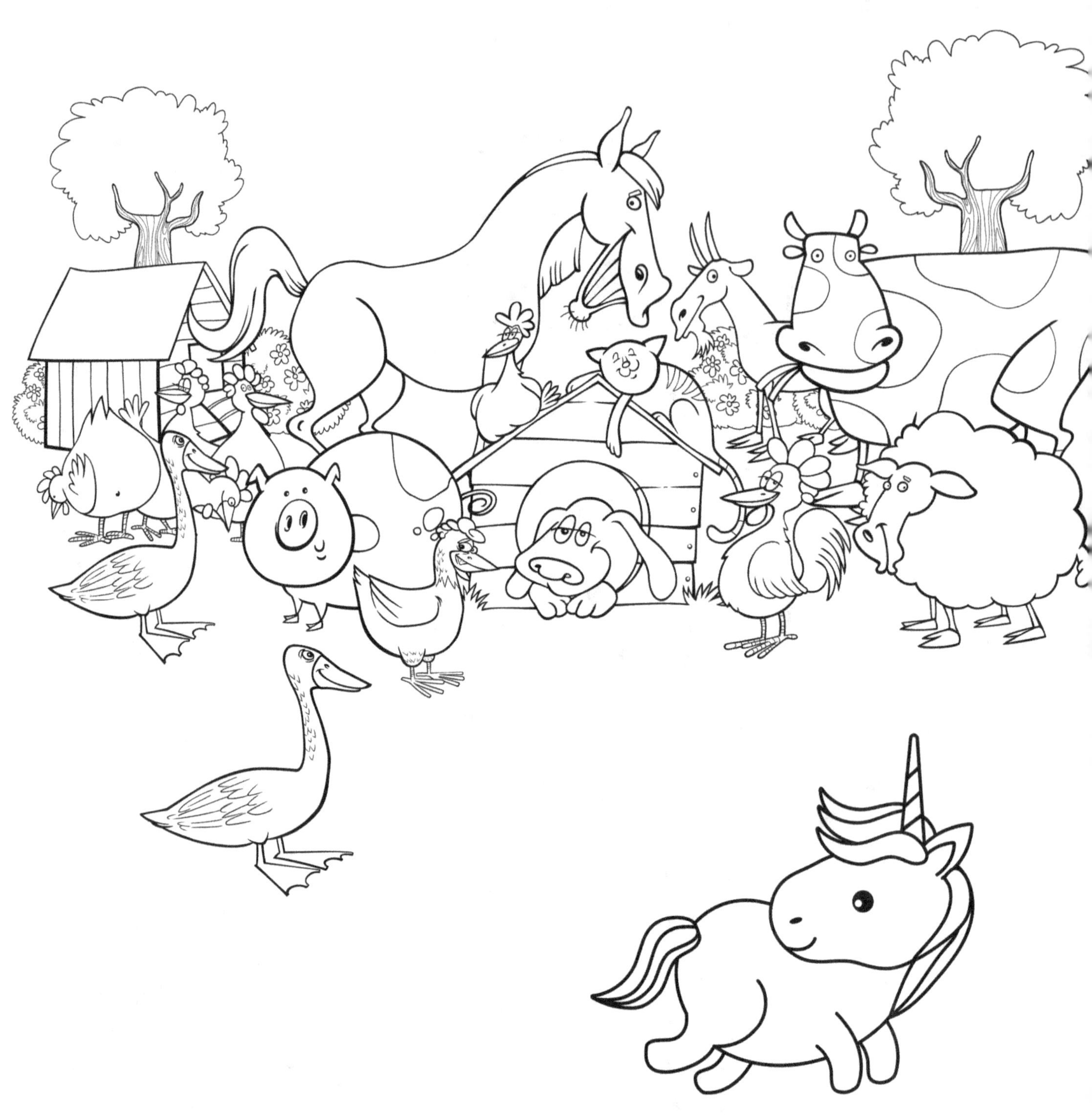

I EVEN LOOKED ON A FARM!

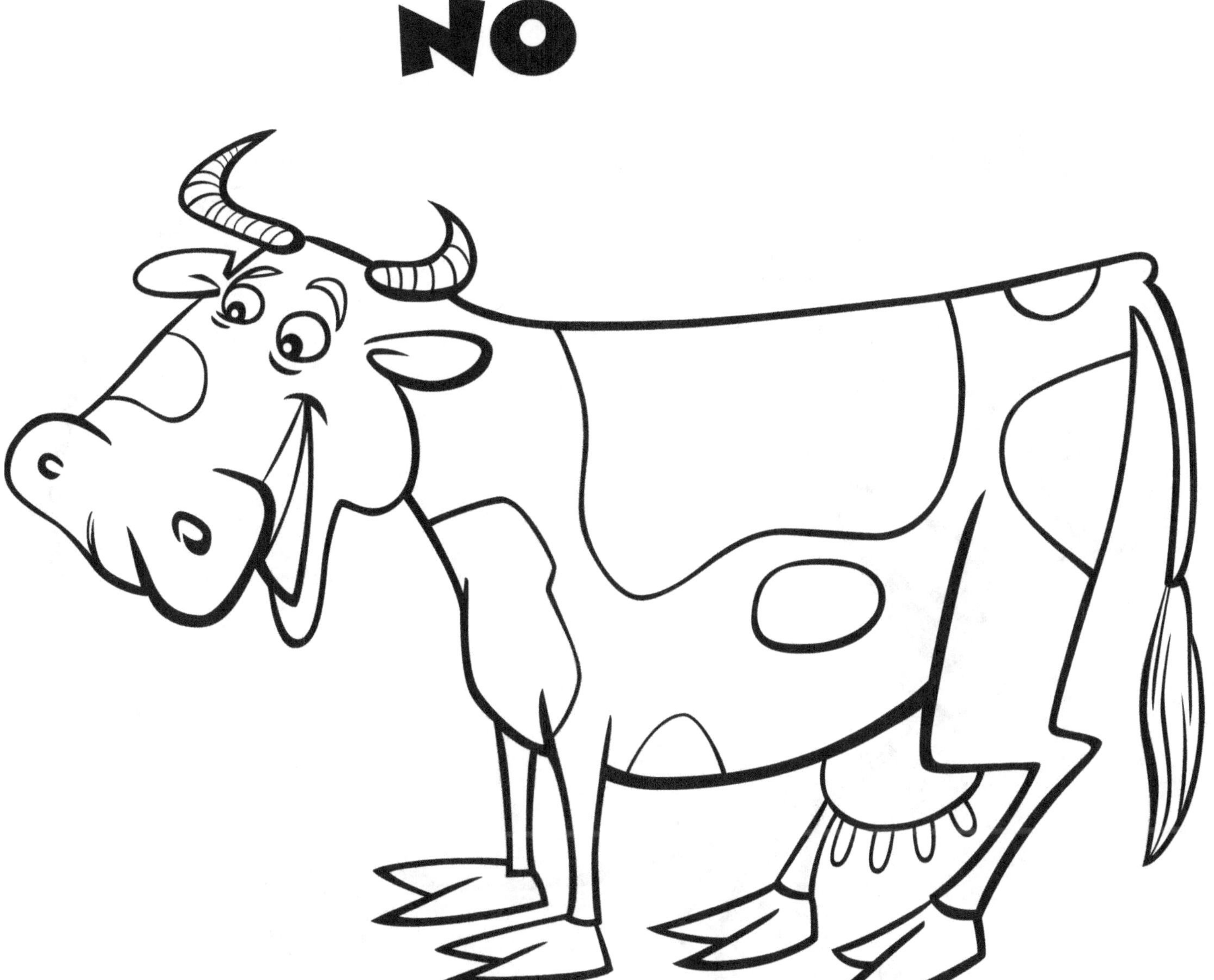

ARE YOU A TYPE 1 DIABETIC?

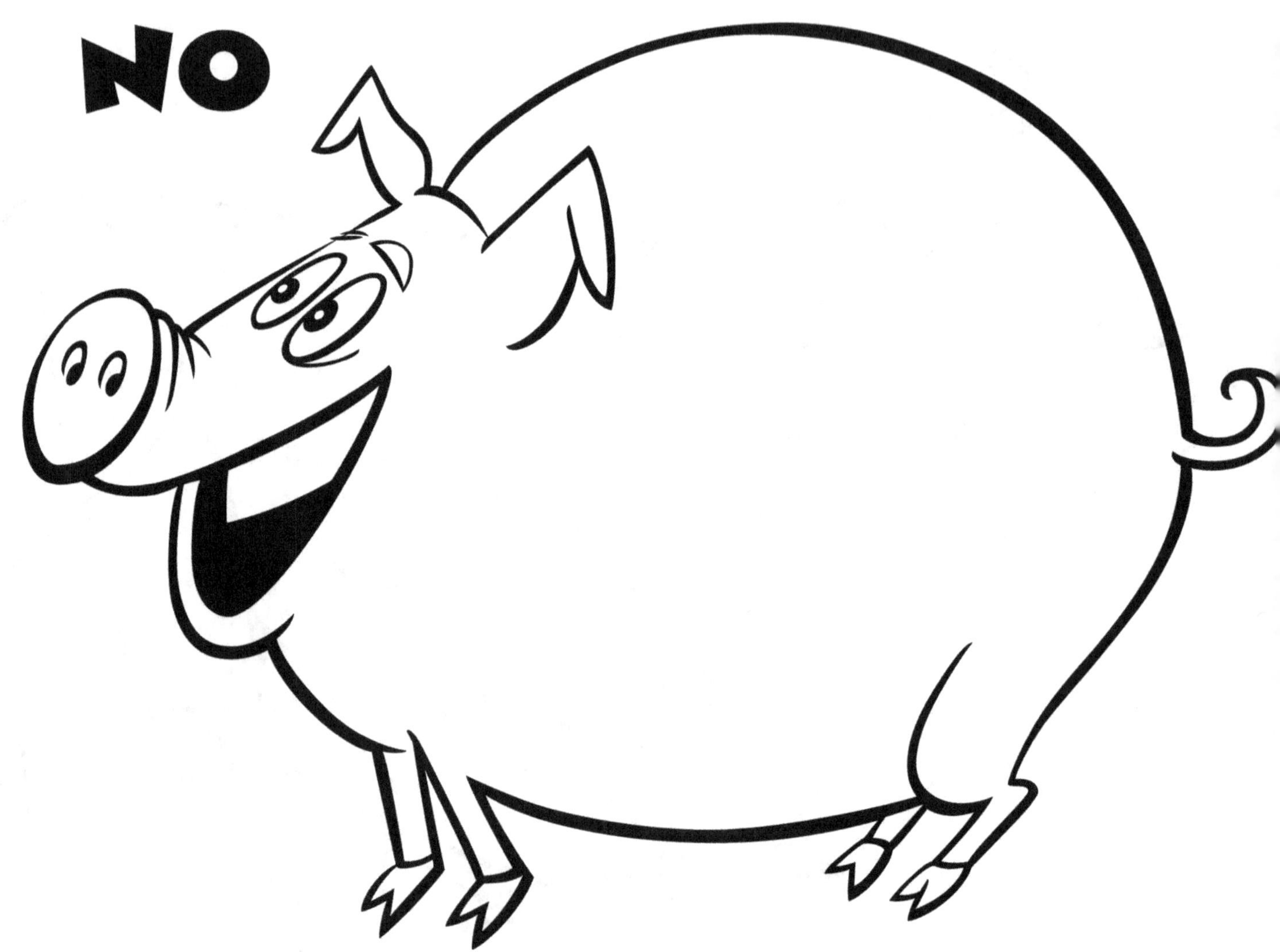

ARE YOU A TYPE 1 DIABETIC?

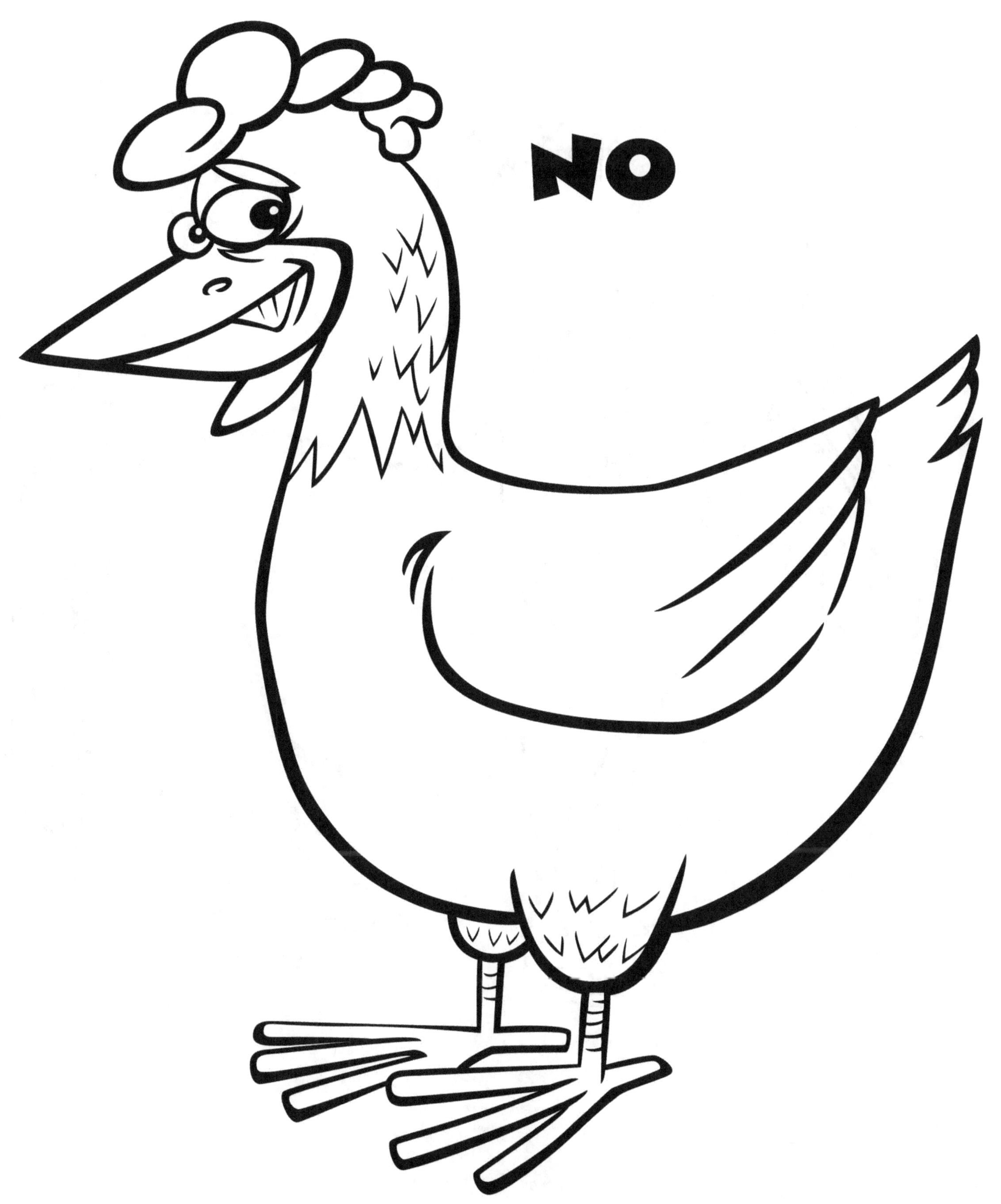

NO
ARE YOU A TYPE 1 DIABETIC?

NO

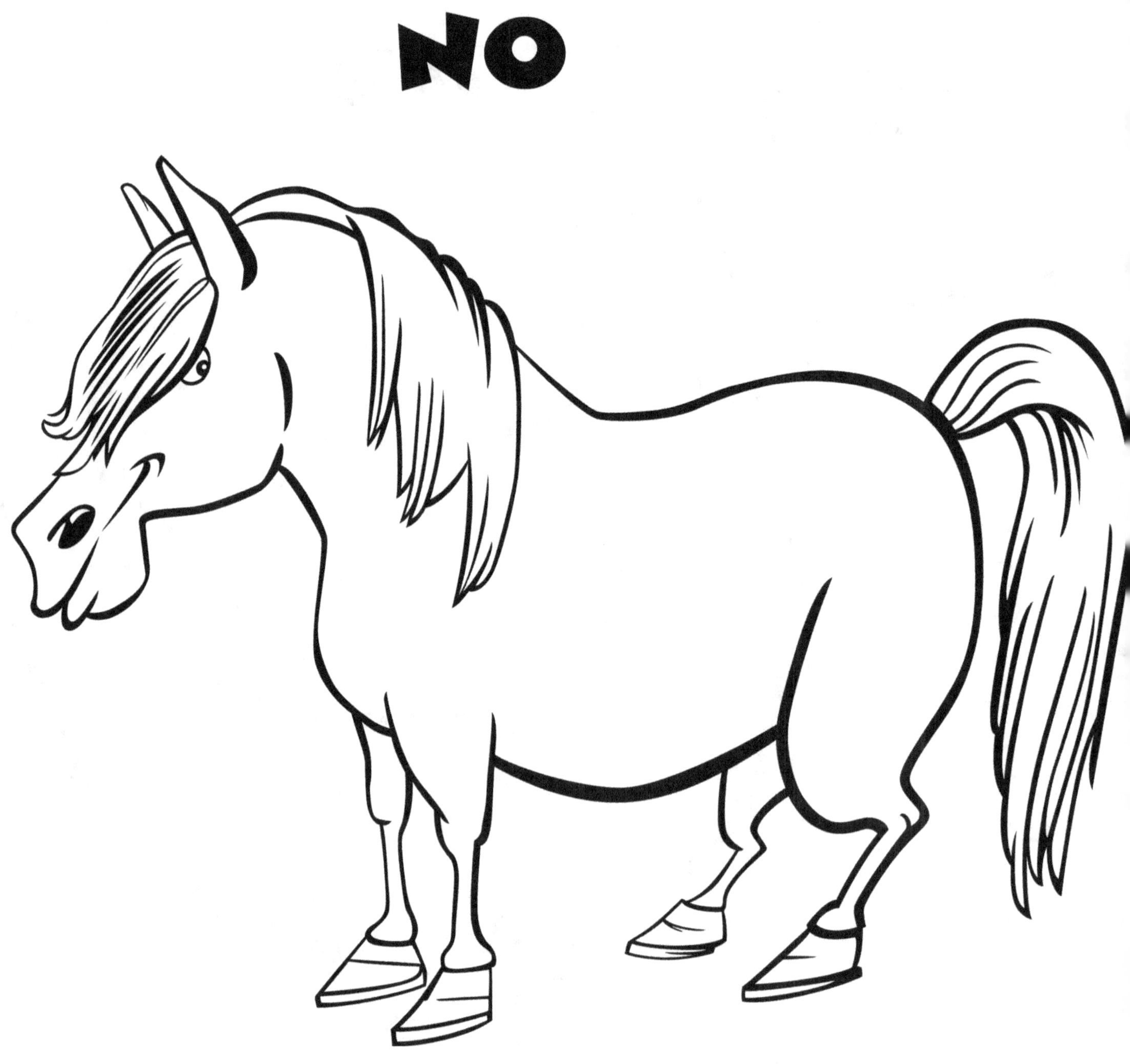

ARE YOU A TYPE 1 DIABETIC.

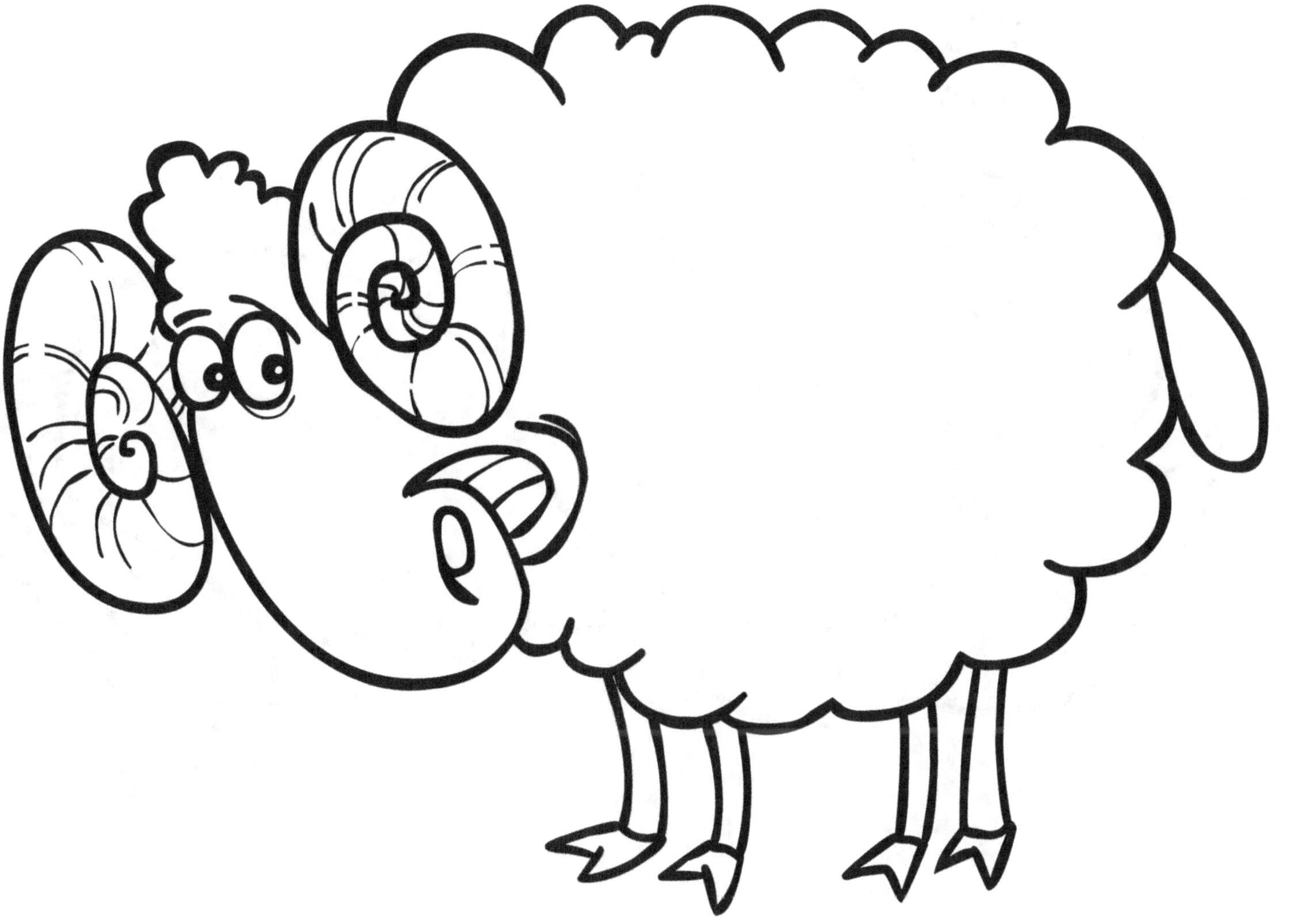

ARE YOU A TYPE 1 DIABETIC?

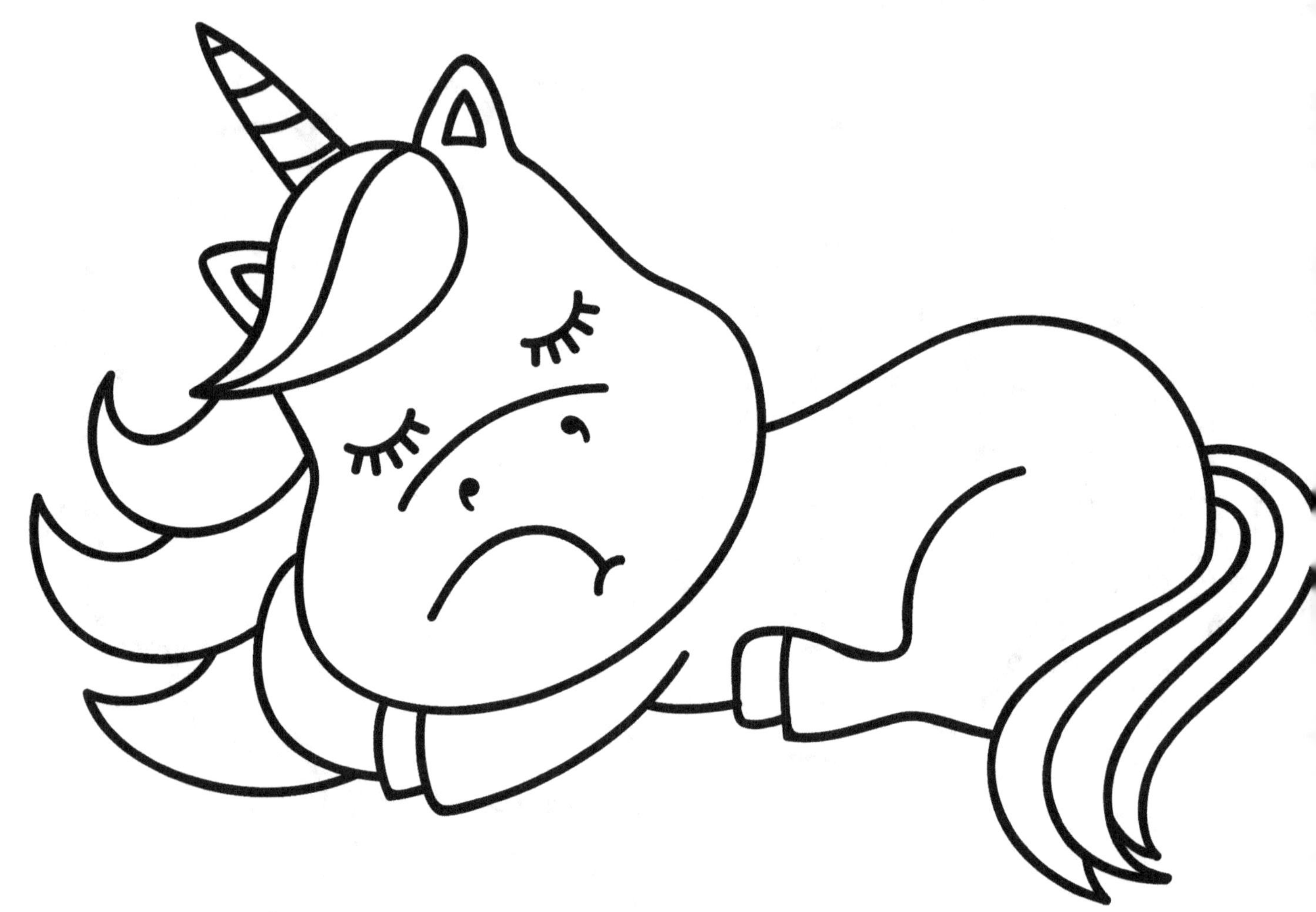

I WAS REALLY SAD
UNTIL ONE DAY....

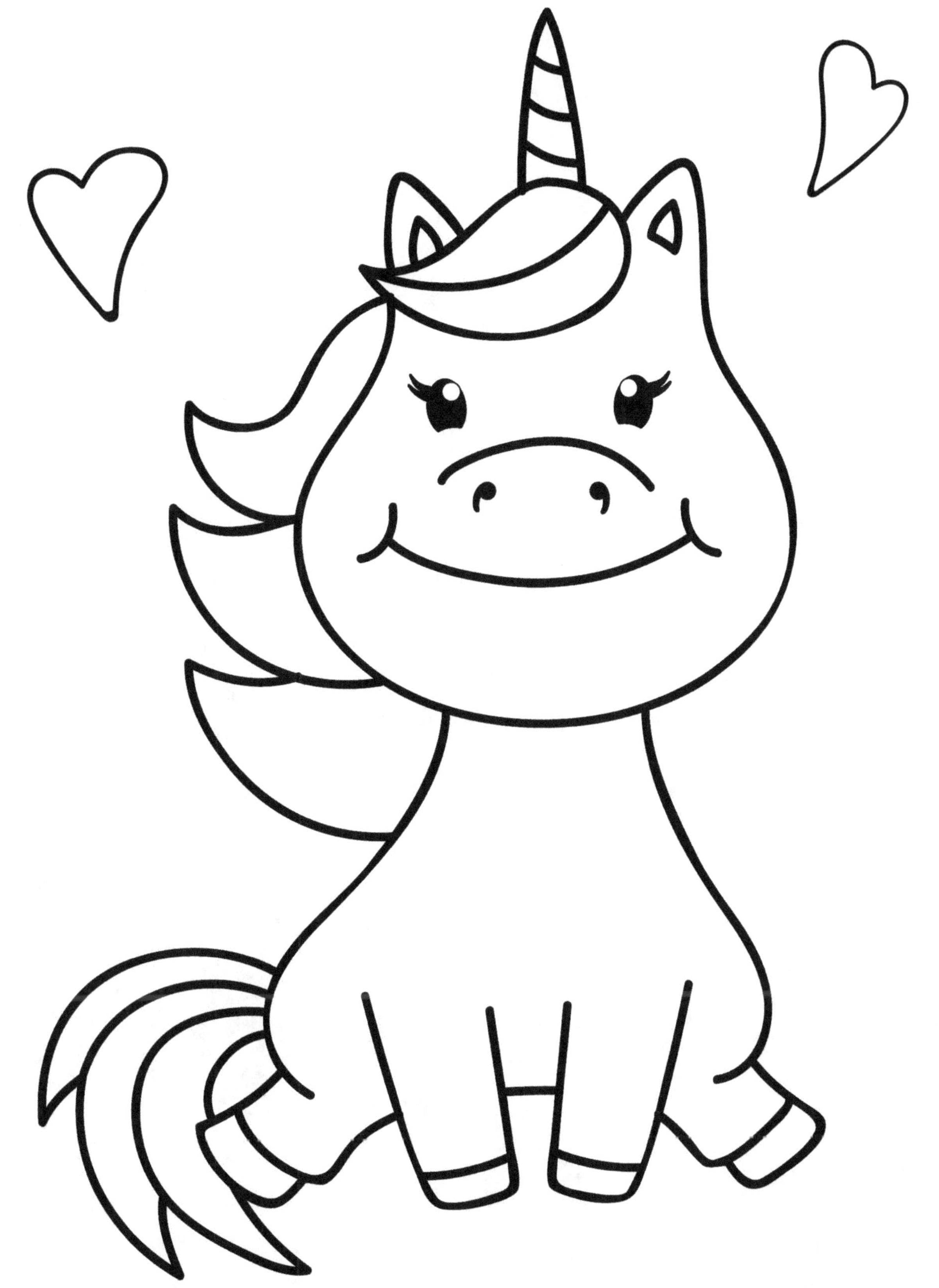

I FOUND MY NEW FRIEND...
YOU!